GW01424248

Check-In time? 5.00pm.

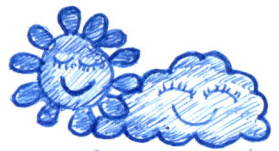

↑

* W4W 05/09/22 *

Change to There is a redeemer → The Wonder of the Cross

Finale! Communion.

↓ * Sced- Ruth * Cor. 3v16.

5 mins

Intro 5mins

2 Songs

Book Review

* Clare Garland
CCTV Wifi?

Printed in Great Britain
by Amazon